Spices, seasonings, and herbs in home cooking

Andrew Collone

Table of Contents

19. Clove

20. Fennel

21. Saffron

22. Garlic

23. Anise

24. Bay leaf

25. Thyme

26. Rosemary

27. Oregano

28. Basil

29. Parsley

30. Cilantro

31. Tarragon

32. Marjoram

33. Mustard

34. Bow

35. Barberry

36. Bergamot

37. Star anise

38. Wasabi

39. Juniper

40. Mint

41. Melissa

42. Dill

43. Chicory

44. Cardamom

45. Cumin

46. Asafetida (ferula)

47. Sage

48. Orange and lemon zest (fresh, dried)

49. Sesame seeds

50. Wild garlic

Book Description

This book is a quick guide to 50 popular food additives. Thanks to them, the products on your table will be even more tasty, rich, and aromatic

01. Salt

Salt a basic seasoning for adding flavor to almost any dish.

Salt is one of the most common and important spices in cooking. It not only imparts the main flavor to dishes, but also helps bring out the flavors of other ingredients. It is used as a preservative, to release flavor, and to regulate moisture in the dough. In addition, salt plays an important role in our body, maintaining the balance of fluids and regulating the nervous system. However, as with other spices, it is important to use it wisely so as not to overdo it and upset the balance of flavors in the dish.

Salt is not considered a spice in the usual sense of the word, as it does not add flavor to dishes, but rather is used to enhance flavor and give balance. However, salt is one of the most important ingredients in cooking and plays a key role in creating the flavor of dishes. It is important to use it in moderation to avoid overdoing it.

Salt enhances the natural taste of products, making them more expressive and rich. It helps create a balance between sweet, sour, bitter, and spicy tastes in dishes. Used for preserving vegetables, meat and fish, helping them preserve for a long time. It is added to meat and poultry marinades to add flavor and help them retain moisture during cooking. Salt is used in recipes for breads, pies, cookies, and other baked goods to even out the flavor and improve texture.

02. Sugar

Sugar can be seen as an ingredient that adds flavor and changes the character of dishes, its effect on the taste and texture of dishes makes it an important component of the culinary arts.

In cooking, sugar is used to create sweet dishes, confectionery, and drinks. It can be used as a single ingredient for sweetening or in combination with other spices to create more complex flavor combinations.

Sugar can also be used in the preparation of various sauces and marinades to add sweetness to dishes and balance the acidity of other ingredients.

Although sugar is usually associated with sweet dishes, its sweetness can also be used to create an interesting balance in many dishes, adding new nuances of flavor.

Sugar can be used to caramelize various ingredients, such as onions, fruits, or vegetables. This gives dishes a sweet-spicy flavor and crunchy texture. Sugar is often added to meat or poultry marinades to give them a sweet taste and help them form an appetizing crust when fried or grilled. In barbecue sauce recipes, sugar is added to balance the acidity of the tomatoes or vinegar and to add a sweet flavor to the sauce. In Asian cuisine, sugar is often added to marinades for pickled vegetables, such as carrots or cucumbers, to impart a sweet and sour flavor. Sugar can be included in various homemade seasonings and mixtures, such as curries or meat rubs, to create a more complex and deeper flavor.

03. Soda

Widely used for household and culinary purposes. For removing odors, as well as for preparing soda water. Baking soda affects the texture and chemical reactions of foods. It has alkaline properties and can be used as an acidifying agent in baking. And also as a leavening agent, helping the dough rise and become more airy. Baking soda can also be used to neutralize acidity in dishessuch as tomato sauces or soups. Soda is used to stew foods.

Sometimes baking soda can be used to soften vegetables before cooking, such as peas or beans, so that they become more tender ore quickly. Its use can be useful for adjusting texture and flavor in some dishes. However, it is important to use it carefully, as too much baking soda can lead to unpleasant-tasting results.

04. Vinegar

An acidic solution produced from the fermentation of alcoholic liquids such as wine, apple juice, or grain alcohol.

It is an unusual but important seasoning in cooking. It adds brightness, acidity, and depth of flavor to dishes.

Vinegar is often used to preserve vegetables, or to marinate meat, poultry, or vegetables, imparting a subtle sour taste and helping them infuse flavors and spices. It can also be added to sauces, salad dressings, soups, and marinades for a richer, richer flavor.

The main types of vinegar are apple cider vinegar, balsamic vinegar, wine vinegar, rice vinegar, etc. Have their own unique characteristics in taste and aroma. They can be used in different dishes to achieve different purposes.

In addition, vinegar can be used to balance the flavor of dishes, especially if they are too sweet or too fatty. Adding a little vinegar can add freshness and character to a dish.

It is important to remember that vinegar is a very concentrated and highly acidic product, so it should be used carefully so as not to overdo it and spoil the taste of the dish

05. Citric acid

Citric acid is an acidic component usually extracted from lemons or other citrus fruits that is widely used in cooking as a flavoring. It adds brightness, acidity, and a refreshing taste to dishes and is also used as a preservative and antioxidant.

Citric acid can be used to add acidity and freshness to a variety of dishes, such as sauces, marinades, salad dressings, canned vegetables, and fruits, and in the production of beverages and desserts.

It is also widely used in canning vegetables and fruits to maintain freshness and brightness of color, as well as to prevent oxidation and preserve nutrients.

Citric acid is a versatile ingredient and can be used alone or in combination with other spices and seasonings to create a variety of flavor profiles. It is important to remember that it is very concentrated, so it should be used carefully so as not to overdo it and change the taste of the dish

06. Starch

Starch plays an important role in cooking and can be used to change the texture and consistency of dishes.

The main function of starch in cooking is as a thickener for sauces, soups, creams, dressings and desserts. It turns liquid ingredients into thickening, giving dishes the desired consistency. Starch also helps prevent the separation of liquid and solid components in dishes, making them more visually appealing.

In addition, starch can be used to make bread mixtures to add a crunchy outer layer to meat, fish, or vegetables when frying or baking.

Some types of starch, such as cornstarch or potato starch, can also serve as a substitute for flour in recipes, making dishes gluten-free or helping to achieve a lighter texture

07. Yeast

Yeast is mainly known as an ingredient in leavening dough and for the production of alcoholic beverages.

Yeast is a microorganism that, when mixed with warm water and sugar, begins to ferment and release carbon dioxide and alcohol, which helps the dough rise and gives baked goods volume and softness.

In addition to its function in rising dough, yeast can also affect the flavor and aroma of baked goods. For example, dry or fresh yeast can add subtle notes of yeasty flavor to bread or cake.

When making bread or other products, yeast can be used along with other seasonings such as salt, sugar, oil, spices, etc. To create a rich flavor and aroma.

08. Gelatin

Gelatin is obtained from collagen found in animal bones, cartilage and skin.

It is used to achieve a certain texture and consistency in dishes. It has the ability to coagulate to form a gel-like mass when cooled, making it a useful ingredient for making jelly-like fillings for cakes, pies, candies, jellies, puddings, marmalade, mousses, and other desserts. It is also used to add density and structure to creams and sauces.

Gelatin can make certain changes in taste characteristics

09. Vanilla

Vanilla is an important culinary herb that adds not only sweetness and aroma, but also depth of flavor to a variety of dishes. This spice has a sweet aroma with notes of caramel and wood.

Vanilla is one of the most popular and recognizable spices used in cooking. Vanilla can be used in a variety of forms, including pods, ground powder, and extract. Vanilla extract is particularly popular and easy to use, as it is easy to dose and adds an intense vanilla flavor to dishes.

Vanilla gives dishes a sweet, aromatic and delicate taste. It is used in a wide range of recipes, from desserts to sweet sauces and drinks. Vanilla flavor can also enhance the flavor of key ingredients in dishes such as milk, eggs or chocolate.

Vanilla has the ability to enhance the flavor of other ingredients and create a deep and rich aroma. It is often used in combination with other spices, such as cinnamon, cloves, or nutmeg, to create complex flavor profiles.

10. Black pepper

Black pepper is one of the most common and versatile spices used in cooking around the world. It is obtained from the fruits of the plant and has a pungent, spicy taste with a slight aroma.

Black pepper can be used either whole or ground. Ground pepper is usually added to dishes before serving or cooking to highlight and enhance the taste of the dish. Whole peppers can be roasted before use to bring out their flavor and heat.

Black pepper is often used to add heat and depth of flavor to various dishes. It is used in the preparation of meat and fish dishes, soups, sauces, marinades, as well as in potato and vegetable dishes. It also perfectly complements the flavors of other spices and seasonings such as cinnamon, cloves, cardamom and ginger.

Apart from its wonderful taste, black pepper also has a number of health benefits. It is considered a natural antioxidant and may help improve digestion and nutrient absorption.

Thus, black pepper is not only an important spice that adds heat and flavor to dishes, but also a useful ingredient for maintaining a healthy lifestyle

11. Red pepper

Cayenne is a spice obtained from the dried fruits of red peppers or hot chili peppers, which has a rich taste and aroma.

Red pepper, or cayenne pepper, is a hot and aromatic type of paper that is widely used in cooking throughout the world. It has a deep red color and a pungent flavor that can range from mild to very spicy, depending on the variety and method of preparation.

Red peppers are often used to add heat and depth of flavor to a variety of dishes. It can be added to sauces, marinades, soups, fried dishes, meat, and vegetable dishes. In addition, red pepper is often used as a main ingredient in seasonings such as chili powder or curry, which add heat and flavor to dishes.

It also has a number of health benefits. Capsicum, an active compound found in red peppers, may help improve overall heart health, speed up metabolism, and reduce inflammation.

Thus, red pepper is an important spice that adds heat and flavor to various dishes and also has several health benefits.

12. Chili pepper

It has a fiery pungency and is often used in Asian, Mexican, and Indian cuisines.

Chili pepper, also known as chili powder or ground red pepper, is one of the most popular and hot spices used in cooking around the world. It is obtained from the dried and ground fruits of various varieties of ground dried red chili peppers.

Chili peppers have a strong, pungent flavor and aroma that can vary greatly depending on the type of pepper and the method of preparation. It is often used to add heat and quaintness to a variety of dishes, such as meat and vegetable dishes, soups, sauces, marinades, condiments, and chili preparations.

Chili pepper can be used as a main spice or added in small quantities to enhance the taste and aroma of dishes. It can also be combined with other spices, such as cumin, coriander, garlic, and oregano, to create complex and rich flavor profiles.

In addition, chili peppers have a number of health benefits. Its active ingredient, capsaicin, may help improve overall heart health, speed up metabolism, reduce appetite, and fight inflammation.

13. Paprika

Paprika is a spice obtained from dried and ground pepper fruits. It has a bright red color and a sweetish aroma with slightly spicy notes. Paprika is often used in cooking to add brightness, color, and flavor to various dishes.

There are several varieties of paprika, including sweet, hot, and smoked. Sweet paprika has a mild and sweet flavor; hot paprika has a spicier and piquant note, and smoked paprika has a rich and deep smoky flavor.

Paprika is widely used in various cuisines around the world. It is often added to goulash, stews, paella, potato dishes, soups, sauces, and marinades, as well as meat and vegetable dishes. Paprika also pairs well with other spices, such as garlic, cumin, coriander, and oregano.

In cooking, paprika not only adds beautiful color and aroma to dishes, but also adds rich flavor and depth. it can also be used as a decoration to give dishes an attractive appearance.

Thus, paprika is an important spice that adds brightness, color, and flavor to various dishes, and also has a variety of flavor options, allowing you to experiment with different culinary styles

14. Cinnamon

Cinnamon is one of the most famous and popular spices, and it is widely used in cooking around the world. Derived from the inner bark of the cinnamon tree, cinnamon has a warm, sweet, and aromatic flavor with slightly spicy notes.

Cinnamon is used in a variety of foods, including desserts, baked goods, drinks, and savory dishes. It is often added to smoothies, coffee, tea, apple pies, muffins, sour shakes, meat marinades, and curries.

This spice is also often used in combination with other spices, such as cloves, nutmeg, and ginger, to create complex flavor profiles in a variety of recipes.

In addition to its culinary uses, cinnamon also has many health benefits. Its properties may include improving digestion, lowering blood sugar, supporting immunity, and having antibacterial and anti-inflammatory properties.

Cinnamon is available in both stick and powder forms. It can also be combined with other spices and ingredients in a variety of recipes to achieve a variety of flavor experiences.

15. Ginger

Ginger is the root of a plant that is widely used as a spice in cooking. It has a sharp and spicy taste, with light citrus and woody notes. Ginger can be used in a variety of forms, including fresh root, powder, syrup, pickles, oils, and others.

In cooking, ginger is added to add aroma and taste to various dishes. It is often used in the preparation of meat and fish dishes, soups, sauces, marinades, baked goods, desserts, drinks, and salad dressings. Ginger also pairs well with other spices, such as garlic, lemongrass, cinnamon, and turmeric, to create a variety of flavor combinations.

In addition, ginger has a number of health benefits. it can help improve digestion, reduce inflammation, soothe the throat, and reduce nausea. Ginger tea is often used to relieve cold symptoms and strengthen the immune system.

16. Turmeric

Turmeric is a spice obtained from the root of the curcuma longa plant, which is part of the ginger family. It has a bright yellow color and a slightly spicy taste, with slight notes of bitterness and citrus.

Turmeric is widely used in cooking, especially in the cuisines of South and Southeast Asia, where it is one of the main spices. it is added to various dishes such as curries, soups, marinades, sauces, rice dishes, desserts and drinks.

Turmeric is also known for its health benefits. It contains an active ingredient called curcumin, which has powerful antioxidant and anti-inflammatory properties. Turmeric may also help improve digestion, support heart health, lower cholesterol, improve brain function, and strengthen the immune system.

Turmeric is usually used in powder form, which is added to dishes as a spice or as an ingredient in various sauces and marinades. It can also be combined with other spices, such as ginger, coriander, cumin, and black pepper, to create complex and rich flavor profiles.

17. Curry

"Curry" is not a single spice, but rather a mixture of various spices that is widely used in cooking, especially in south and southeast Asian countries. The composition of curry may vary depending on region and preference, but usually includes spices such as turmeric, coriander, cumin, ginger, cardamom, cinnamon, cloves, chili pepper, etc.

Curry powder, often called simply "curry," is a mixture of these spices in certain proportions. it has a variety of flavors, usually bright and aromatic, with a slight spicy note and hints of sweetness.

Curry is used to prepare a variety of dishes, including meat and vegetable curries, rice curries, curry soups, and many others. It gives dishes a rich taste and aroma and also adds a beautiful yellow or orange color.

Curry is also a very flexible spice that can be adapted to suit different taste preferences and dietary restrictions. It can be spicy or sweet, depending on the spices used and the amount of chili pepper.

Thus, curry is a multifunctional and versatile spice that adds flavor and aroma to a variety of dishes and also allows you to experiment with different flavor profiles and culinary styles.

18. Nutmeg

Nutmeg is a spice obtained from the seeds of the fruit of the nutmeg tree (myristica fragranta). It has a sweet, warm, and rich aroma with light spicy and woody notes.

Nutmeg is often used in cooking to prepare a variety of dishes, including sweet and savory. It is added to dough for pies, cakes, muffins, buns, and cream sauces, as well as to various meat, fish and vegetable dishes. Nutmeg can also be used in combination with other spices, such as cinnamon, cloves, ginger, and cardamom to create complex flavor profiles.

However, it is important to remember that nutmeg should be used with care and restraint, as its strong flavor can dominate dishes. In small quantities, it gives dishes a pleasant and rich taste, but in large quantities, it can become too spicy and even bitter.

Apart from its culinary uses, nutmeg also has some health benefits. Its oil and extract may help improve digestion, reduce stress, improve sleep, and have antibacterial and anti-inflammatory properties.

Thus, nutmeg is an important and versatile spice that adds warmth, aroma and rich flavor to a variety of dishes.

19. Clove

Cloves are a spice obtained from the dried flower buds of the clove tree (syzygium aromaticum). it has a rich aroma and spicy taste with light sweet and woody notes.

Cloves are often used in cooking to prepare various dishes, both sweet and savory. It is added to potato dishes, marinades, soups, sauces, seasonings, baked goods, and various meat and fish dishes. Cloves are also often found in spice blends such as curry, garam masala, and Punjabi masala.

In cooking, cloves have not only a spicy aroma, but also antiseptic properties, so they can also be added to dishes that require preservation or long-term storage.

In addition to their culinary uses, cloves may also have health benefits. It can help improve digestion, reduce inflammation, relieve pain and cough, and strengthen the immune system.

Cloves are available as whole buds or in ground form. It can also be combined with other spices, such as cinnamon, cardamom, nutmeg, and ginger, to create complex and rich flavor profiles.

20. Fennel

Fennel is a plant whose parts are used as a spice in cooking. It is known for its light, sweet aroma and taste, which are reminiscent of anise. Fennel can be used in a variety of forms, including seeds, leaves, and roots.

Fennel seeds are the most common form of this spice and are widely used in cooking. they add aroma and flavor to a variety of dishes, including soups, sauces, marinades, salads, meat and fish dishes. Fennel seeds are also often used in baking and as a seasoning for bread and cheese.

Fennel also has some health benefits. Its seeds are known for their carminative properties, which can help improve digestion and relieve bloating. Fennel also contains antioxidants and other nutrients that may be beneficial for heart health, the immune system, and overall well-being.

In cooking, fennel has versatile uses and can be used as a spice on its own or in combination with other ingredients to create a variety of flavor profiles. Its moderately sweet aroma makes it especially suitable for dishes containing meat, poultry, fish, vegetables, and cheeses.

21. Saffron

Saffron is one of the most expensive and luxurious spices in the world, obtained from crocus flowers (Crocus sativus). It has a bright yellow or orange color and an intense aroma. Saffron is usually sold in the form of small red threads known as "saffron threads.".

Saffron is widely used in cooking to add bright color, aroma, and taste to dishes. It is often added to rice dishes, sauces, soups, paella, desserts, baked goods, and various meat and fish dishes. Saffron is also a key ingredient in dishes such as biryani and risotto.

Moreover, saffron also has a number of health benefits. Its active components, including croqueting and saffron, have antioxidant, anti-inflammatory, and antibacterial properties. Safflower can also help improve your mood, reduce stress, and relieve cold symptoms.

However, it is worth noting that saffron is a very expensive product due to its complex production process. It is handpicked from crocus flowers and requires many flowers to produce a small amount of the spice. It is because of this that saffron is considered a luxurious and prestigious spice.

Thus, saffron is a luxurious and unique spice that adds brightness, aroma, and taste to various dishes, and also has several health benefits.

22. Garlic

Garlic is a plant from the lily family. Onion slices ("cloves") are eaten raw or cooked. Leaves, arrows, and peduncles are also edible and are used mainly on young plants. It has a strong aroma and a sharp, rich taste.

Garlic is often used in cooking to add aroma and flavor to dishes. It is added to various soups, sauces, marinades, salad dressings, meat and vegetable dishes, pizza, pasta, and much more. Garlic can also be used to create garlic oil and garlic powder, which are also widely used in cooking.

In addition, garlic has many health benefits. Its active components, such as allicin, have antibacterial, antioxidant, and anti-inflammatory properties. Garlic may also help lower blood cholesterol, improve blood circulation, support the immune system, and even reduce the risk of certain diseases, such as heart disease and some types of cancer.

23. Anise

Anise is a spice obtained from the fruit of the plant Campanella anisum, which belongs to the Apiaceae family. It has a sweetish aroma and taste, with light notes of licorice and spice.

Anise is often used in cooking to add aroma and flavor to various dishes. Its seeds can be added to baked goods, cookies, muffins, cakes, and ice cream, as well as various drinks such as mulled wine, hot chocolate, tea, and coffee. Anise is also often found in various spices and spice blends, such as curry, garam masala, and anise salt.

In addition to its use in cooking, anise also has a number of health benefits. Its seeds contain anethole, which is the active component of anise and has antibacterial, anti-inflammatory, and antiviral properties. Anise may also help improve digestion, relieve gas and bloating, and relieve coughs and sore throats.

Anise can be used as a spice on its own or in combination with other ingredients to create a variety of flavor profiles. Its sweet aroma and taste make it especially suitable for making desserts and drinks.

Thus, anise is an important and versatile spice that adds aroma and flavor to a variety of dishes, as well as having health benefits

24. Bay leaf

Bay leaf is a spice obtained from the bay tree (Taurus nobilis), which belongs to the grape family. Bay leaf has an intense aroma with light spicy notes and a bitter taste.

Bay leaves are often used in cooking to add aroma and flavor to various dishes. It is added to soups, sauces, marinades, stews, broths, canned vegetables, and meat dishes. Bay leaves are also often used when cooking rice to add aroma and flavor.

Besides their use in cooking, bay leaves also have a number of health benefits. Its active components, such as eucalyptus and kineol, have antiseptic and anti-inflammatory properties. Bay leaf can also help improve digestion and relieve symptoms of gas and bloating.

Bay leaves are usually added to dishes as whole leaves, which are then removed before serving. It can also be ground and used in spice blends to add aroma and flavor to a variety of dishes.

Thus, bay leaf is an important and versatile spice that adds aroma and flavor to a variety of dishes, as well as having health benefits

25. Thyme

Thyme is an aromatic herbal plant with small leaves, belonging to the genus Thymus. Thyme has a strong, spicy aroma and taste with light citrus undertones.

Thyme is widely used in a variety of dishes, including meat, fish, vegetables, soups, sauces, salad dressings, and baked goods. It is often used as a seasoning for dishes such as poultry, fish, and vegetables, as well as in sauces, marinades, and soups. Thyme can also be used fresh or dried, depending on the recipe and preference.

Besides its use in cooking, thyme is also known for its medicinal properties. It contains many beneficial compounds, such as flavonoids, tannins, and essential oils,,,, that can help manage inflammation, improve digestion, reduce stress, strengthen the immune system, and even help with colds.

Thyme also contains antimicrobial properties that make it useful in fighting bacteria and other microorganisms. Some cultures even use it to preserve food.

26. Rosemary

Rosemary is an evergreen shrub with needle-shaped leaves and aromatic flowers that are used in cooking to add aroma and flavor to dishes. Rosemary has a strong, spicy, piney flavor with light citrus notes and an aroma with woody and herbal undertones.

Rosemary is widely used in various dishes, such as meat, fish, vegetables, pasta, potatoes, and baked and grilled dishes. It can also be added to marinades, sauces, soups, salad dressings, and baked goods. Rosemary has the ability to add a deep and rich flavor to dishes.

Besides its culinary uses, rosemary is also known for its health benefits. It contains antioxidants such as consul and Rosmarie acid, which can help protect the body from free radical damage and prevent oxidative stress. Additionally, rosemary may also help improve digestion, support heart health, reduce stress levels, and improve memory and concentration.

Rosemary can be used either fresh or dried. It can be added whole to dishes or ground before use. Rosemary leaves are also often used to create incense sticks and oils, which can add aroma and flavor to a variety of foods and drinks

27. Oregano

Oregano is a herbal plant with small leaves and fragrant flowers. Oregano has a strong and warm aroma, and its taste is sweet with light spicy notes.

Oregano is often used in various dishes, such as Italian cuisine, pizza, pasta, soups, salads, marinades, and meat and fish dishes. It can also be added to olive oil to create a flavorful sauce or used as a seasoning for popcorn and potatoes. Oregano has the ability to give dishes a rich and aromatic taste.

Besides its culinary uses, oregano is also known for its health benefits. It contains antioxidants and flavonoids, which can help protect the body from free radical damage and improve the immune system. Oregano may also help improve digestion, reduce inflammation, and have antimicrobial properties.

Oregano is usually used in its dried form, although fresh leaves can also be used. It can be added to dishes at the beginning of cooking or used as a seasoning before serving. It can also be mixed with other spices such as basil, thyme, and rosemary to create complex flavor profiles

28. Basil

Basil is an aromatic herbal plant with oval leaves that have a sweet taste and a pleasant aroma. Basil has a sweetish taste with light, spicy, and herbal notes and an aroma with mint, citrus and herbal undertones.

Basil is widely used in various dishes, especially in Italian cuisine. It is often added to pastas, pizza, soups, salads, sauces, marinades, and many other dishes. Basil is also a key ingredient in the popular pesto sauce. It has the ability to give dishes a fresh and aromatic taste.

Besides its use in cooking, basil is also known for its health benefits. It contains antioxidants such as vitamin K and flavonoids, which can help protect the body from free radical damage and improve heart health. Basil may also help improve digestion, reduce inflammation, and have antimicrobial properties.

Basil is usually used fresh, but it can also be dried. It can be added to dishes at the beginning of cooking or used as a seasoning before serving. It can also be mixed with other spices, such as oregano, thyme, and rosemary, to create complex flavor profiles.

29. Parsley

Parsley is a herbal plant with serrated leaves and tender stems that have a fresh taste and aroma. Parsley has a fresh, light taste with herbal and citrus notes and an aroma with spicy and herbal undertones.

Parsley can be used as a decoration for dishes or as an ingredient for preparing various dishes. It is often added to salads, soups, sauces, marinades, pickles, vegetables, and meat dishes. Parsley is also a key ingredient in many national cuisines. It has the ability to give dishes a fresh and aromatic taste.

Apart from its culinary uses, parsley is also known for its health benefits. It contains many vitamins, minerals, and antioxidants that can help strengthen the immune system, improve digestion, and have anti-inflammatory properties.

Parsley is usually used fresh, but it can also be dried. It can be added to dishes at the beginning of cooking or used as a seasoning before serving. Parsley can also be mixed with other spices, such as dill, basil, and oregano, to create complex flavor profiles.

30. Cilantro

Cilantro, also known as coriander, It is a herbal plant with delicate, serrated leaves and aromatic stems that taste fresh and aromatic. Cilantro has a distinctive, fresh citrus aroma.

Cilantro can be used fresh or dried, and its leaves can be added to dishes at the beginning or end of cooking. Leaves are added to salads, soups, salad dressings, marinades, and many other dishes. The leaves are also used to decorate dishes and give them a fresh and aromatic taste.

Cilantro seeds can be ground before use or added whole and can be added to a variety of dishes, including marinades, sauces, and baked goods. It is also often used in spice blends such as curries and garam masala to add more complex flavor profiles to dishes.

Apart from its culinary uses, cilantro is also known for its health benefits. It contains vitamins, minerals, and antioxidants that can help strengthen the immune system, improve digestion, and have anti-inflammatory properties. Additionally, cilantro may help lower cholesterol and improve heart health.

31. Tarragon

Tarragon, also known as tarragon, is a herbal plant with narrow leaves and aromatic stems that have a sweet, slightly sour taste and a strong, pleasant aroma.

Tarragon is commonly used in salads, sauces, marinades, vinegars, soups, and many other dishes. It is often added to meat, fish, and vegetable dishes to give them a rich aroma and taste. Tarragon is also a key ingredient in the classic French béarnaise sauce and Russian tarragon vinegar.

Besides its culinary uses, tarragon is also known for its health benefits. It contains vitamins, minerals, and antioxidants that can help strengthen the immune system, improve digestion, and have anti-inflammatory properties. Tarragon may also help lower blood sugar and have antimicrobial properties.

Tarragon can be used either fresh or dried. It can be added to dishes at the beginning of cooking or used as a seasoning before serving. Tarragon can also be mixed with other spices, such as parsley, basil, and dill, to create complex flavor profiles.

32. Marjoram

Marjoram is aherbal plant with small leaves and tender stems from the Lauraceae family. Marjoram has a spicy taste with the aroma of mint and herbs, with herbal undertones.

Marjoram is often added to various dishes, such as meat, fish, vegetables, soups, sauces, and marinades. It is used both fresh and dried. Marjoram gives dishes a rich aroma and taste, especially meat and vegetable dishes. It is also a key ingredient in many spice blends, such as herbs and spices.

Besides its use in cooking, marjoram is also known for its health benefits. It contains vitamins, minerals, and antioxidants that can help strengthen the immune system, improve digestion, and have anti-inflammatory properties. Marjoram may also help reduce stress levels and relieve some allergy symptoms.

Marjoram is usually added to dishes at the beginning of cooking or as a seasoning before serving. Dried marjoram has a stronger flavor than fresh marjoram. It can also be mixed with other spices to create complex flavor combinations

33. Mustard

Mustard is a spice made from the seeds of the mustard plant, a calciferous plant. Mustard seeds can be used whole or ground to create mustard paste or powder, which is then mixed with liquid (most often vinegar or water) to create ready-made mustard.

Mustard adds spiciness and a characteristic aroma to dishes. It is often used in cooking to add flavor and aroma to meat and fish dishes, sauces, marinades, salad dressings, canned vegetables, and marinades. Mustard can also be used in baking to add a tangy flavor to breads or pies.

In addition, mustard has antimicrobial and antioxidant properties and also contains vitamins and minerals such as magnesium and selenium, which are beneficial for health.

There are several types of mustard, including regular mustard (yellow mustard) and Dijon mustard, which have different flavors and spiciness. For example, Dijon mustard has a sharper flavor and smoother texture than regular mustard.

Mustard can also be used as a base ingredient to create various sauces and marinades, as well as to marinate meat before cooking.

Thus, mustard is not only a spice that adds heat and flavor to dishes, but also a healthy ingredient with antimicrobial and antioxidant properties

34. Bow

Onions are not only a common vegetable, but also an important seasoning that is widely used in cooking around the world. It adds a spicy-hot taste to various dishes and also gives them a characteristic aroma and piquancy. Onions can be used either fresh, dried, or powdered.

Fresh onions can be used to prepare various dishes, such as soups, sauces, marinades, salads, meat dishes, and vegetable dishes. It can be added at the beginning of cooking or used as an additional seasoning before serving. Fresh onions have a pungent taste and aroma that will add brightness and richness to the dish.

Dried onions are also widely used in cooking. It can be added to soups, sauces, salad dressings, cooked dishes, and marinades. Dried onions have a milder taste compared to fresh ones, but they retain their characteristic aroma and give the dish a special taste.

Onions can also be used in the form of onion powder, which is added to various dishes to add aroma and taste. Onion powder can be used as a main ingredient in many dishes, including soups, sauces, marinades, and seasonings.

35. Barberry

Barberry is the fruit of a shrub that grows mainly in temperate climates. Barberry fruits have a sour taste and are used in cooking to add sourness and flavor. Barberry is not as popular a spice as some other herbs and spices, but its sweet and sour berries can be used to prepare a variety of dishes and drinks.

Barberry berries contain acids, including citric and malice. They can be used in the preparation of preserves, jams, compotes, juices, sauces, and seasonings for meat. They can also be added to baked goods, salads, and omelet's to add acidity and brightness.

Barberry is also often used in traditional Chinese cuisine, where the berries are added to a variety of dishes, including fried rice dishes, soups and sauces, to impart a sweet and sour flavor.

In addition, barberry can be used to prepare an aromatic drink known as barberry tea. To do this, the berries are boiled in water along with other herbs and spices, such as ginger and cinnamon, to create an aromatic and delicious drink.

36. Bergamot

Bergamot is a citrus fruit whose fruits are used to obtain aromatic oils as well as to be eaten as zest or added to drinks.

Bergamot is widely known as a source of aromatic oils that are used in perfumes and cosmetic products. However, in cooking, bergamot can also be used as a spice.

This citrus fruit, known for its bright aroma and sweet and sour taste, can be added to various dishes to add a special taste. Usually, bergamot is used in the form of a peel or drops of oil. Its peel can be used to make aromatic syrups, add to baked goods, prepare desserts, or flavor meat and fish dishes. Bergamot oil can also be used to flavor various dishes, drinks, or even as a base for sauces and marinades.

Bergamot has a bright citrus flavor with notes of lemon, orange and lime. It gives dishes a special freshness and aroma, making them more refined and attractive.

However, it is worth noting that using bergamot in cooking should be done with caution, as it can be quite intense to use. A small amount of bergamot can add a pleasant aroma and taste to a dish, but too much can lead to an overabundance of citrus notes and bitterness.

Thus, bergamot, although not the most common spice in cooking, can be an interesting and original way to add aroma and flavor to various dishes

37. Star anise

Star anise It is an aromatic spice that is widely used in cooking, especially in Asian and Arabic cuisines. Star anise has a rich, bright anise aroma with tart notes and a sweetish taste.

Can be used as whole stars or ground powder. Star anise is often added to marinades, sauces, soups, meat, and fish dishes, as well as baked goods and desserts. It is also a key ingredient in many spice mixtures, such as Chinese powder.

In addition to its use in cooking, star anise also has a number of health benefits. It contains antioxidants and essential oils that may help improve digestion, reduce inflammation, and have antimicrobial properties. Star anise is also used in traditional medicine to relieve cold symptoms, reduce abdominal pain, and relieve stress.

Star anise is usually added to dishes at the beginning of cooking or as a seasoning before serving. It can be used either alone or with other spices

38. Wasabi

Wasabi is the pungent and aromatic root of the wasabi Maponics plant, and is widely used as a seasoning in Japanese cuisine. In appearance, it resembles horseradish but has a milder taste and a more complex aroma.

Wasabi is usually served as a green paste or powder that is diluted with water to form a paste. It is often used as a seasoning for sushi, sashimi, rolls, and other Japanese dishes. Wasabi adds a spicy, refreshing flavor to dishes, making it a popular addition to seafood and raw fish.

Wasabi root contains isothiocyanates, which give it its pungency and specific taste. In addition, wasabi has antimicrobial properties and can help fight bacteria in food.

Wasabi can also be used as a seasoning for meat and vegetable dishes, as well as for sauces and marinades. It can also be added to salad dressings to add zest and flavor.

In cooking, wasabi is often mixed with soy sauce to create wasabi soy sauce, which complements sushi and sashimi

39. Juniper

Juniper is a spice obtained from the berries of the juniper tree, which is a coniferous shrub. Juniper berries have a special aroma and taste, and they are widely used in cooking to flavor various dishes.

Juniper berries can be used fresh, dried, or ground. They are often added to meat dishes such as beef, lamb, pork, and poultry to add rich aroma and flavor. Juniper is also widely used in the preparation of salty foods, including pickling vegetables and marinating meats.

In cooking, juniper is also used to flavor alcoholic beverages such as gin and various bitters and liqueurs. Juniper berries can be added to cocktails and martinis to add a unique aroma and taste.

In addition, juniper can be used as a seasoning for preparing various dishes, including sauces, marinades, soups, salads and even baked goods. It has a light citrus and pine aroma that can add a distinct and unique flavor to dishes.

However, it is worth remembering that juniper berries have a rather strong aroma, so they should be used with caution so as not to overdo the quantity. In large quantities, juniper can give a dish a bitter taste

40. Mint

Mint is a herbal plant with aromatic leaves that have a fresh and cool taste and are widely used in cooking and beverages.

Mint is often used in the preparation of various dishes and drinks, as well as in the home pharmacy. It has a refreshing taste and aroma that goes well with many ingredients.

Mint can be used either fresh or dried. Its leaves are added to salads, soups, sauces, marinades, drinks, and desserts to give them a refreshing taste and aroma. Mint also goes well with fruits, vegetables, meat, fish, and seafood.

In cooking, mint is often used in dishes such as Thai salad, lemonade, mint tea, mint ice cream, mint sauce and much more. It is also added to various cocktails and marinades.

Thus, mint not only has a refreshing taste and aroma but can also be used as a spice for preparing various dishes and drinks.

41. Melissa

Lemon balm is an aromatic herb plant with a lemony aroma and minty notes that is often used in cooking and medicine.

It is used as an aromatic spice in the sense that its leaves can be added to dishes to impart a unique taste and aroma. It goes well with fish, poultry, seafood, and vegetables.

Lemon balm can be used in soups, salads, marinades, sauces, and desserts. Its leaves can also be added to drinks to impart a refreshing lemon flavor and aroma.

Although lemon balm is not as common in cooking as some other spices, its unique lemony flavor and aroma can add an interesting and refreshing twist to dishes.

42. Dill

Dill is an aromatic herbal plant with small green leaves and a strong aroma and taste that is widely used in cooking to flavor various dishes. Its fresh taste and aroma can greatly enhance the taste of the dish.

Dill has a fresh, light aroma with light citrus notes and a slight anise aroma. It is often added to dishes in the last moments of cooking or even before serving to maintain its fresh taste and aroma.

Dill is often used in salads, soups, sauces, and marinades. It also goes well with seafood, potatoes, cucumbers and young vegetables. Dill seeds can be used as a seasoning for smoked meat, marinades, and fish dishes.

43. Chicory

Chicory is a root vegetable of the plant that is dried, roasted and used as a coffee substitute or added to various dishes to impart a distinctive taste and aroma.

Chicory has a bitter taste and can add interesting notes to a variety of dishes. Its powder or crushed roots are used to flavor pies, muffins, soups, sauces, marinades, and other dishes.

In cooking, chicory can be used either alone or in combination with other spices. For example, it can be added to spice mixtures to add depth of flavor and aroma. Chicory can also be used in drinks, such as coffee, to add a bitter flavor.

44. Cardamom

Cardamom is the seed of the fruit of the altar cardamom plant, which is part of the ginger plant family. It is one of the most popular and widely used spices in cooking. Cardamom has a sweetish, spicy taste with light citrus notes and a strong aroma.

Cardamom can be used either as whole grains or in ground form. It gives dishes a special taste and aroma, making them more interesting and rich.

Cardamom is added to many dishes in various cuisines, including Indian, Arabic, and Scandinavian. It is used in marinades, sauces, soups, curries, and meat dishes. Added to hot drinks such as coffee, tea, mulled wine, and milk tea to add flavor. Often added to dough, various desserts, including ice cream and puddings

45. Cumin

Cuminhas a warm, spicy taste with tart and sweet notes and an aroma with light citrus undertones.

Cumin can be used in the form of whole seeds or ground powder. It imparts an intense aroma and rich flavor to dishes, making them more appealing to your palate.

Widely used in Asian, Indian, Mexican and Mediterranean cuisines.

Cumin is ideal for meat dishes such as beef, lamb, chicken, and fish. It can be added to marinades, bean dishes, and salads.

Goes well with vegetables such as potatoes, carrots, broccoli and cauliflower.

Cumin is one of the key ingredients for preparing pilaf and other rice dishes.

Can be added to the dough for bread, pies, cookies, and other baked goods.

46. Asafetida (ferula)

Asafetida, also known as "devil's scented powder", is a resin from the roots and rhizomes of the ferula plant, which has a very strong and unpleasant odor when raw, but when cooked it takes on more pleasant notes. Reminiscent of garlic and onions.

Asafetida is a key ingredient in Indian, Iranian, Pakistani, and Afghani cuisines. It is added to various dishes, such as pilaf, couscous, and meat dishes.

Goes well with legume dishes such as lentils, chickpeas and beans. It is added when cooking beans to improve their taste and reduce gas formation.

Asafetida can be added to sauces, marinades and salad dressings to add depth of flavor and aroma.

In some cultures, asafetida is also used for medicinal purposes, as a remedy for gas and stomach upsets.

It is important to remember that asafetida has a strong and rather specific taste and smell, so it should be used with caution when adding small amounts to dishes.

47. Sage

Sage is an herbaceous plant with silvery leaves and an aroma and taste that resembles mint and camphor, and is used in cooking and medicine.

Spicy and tart taste with the aroma of mint and camphor. The scent is aromatic and refreshing.

Sage goes well with meat, fish, and baked goods. It can be added to marinades, soups, sauces, stews, and salad dressings.

Can be added to marinades and brines for preserving vegetables and fruits. It adds aroma and flavor to them and helps extend their shelf life

48. Orange and lemon zest (fresh, dried)

Orange and lemon peel is the peel or outer covering of oranges or lemons that contains many essential oils and aromatic compounds. Usually, the zest is used to give dishes a bright citrus aroma and taste.

The zest is used to flavor baked goods, desserts, confectionery, cocktails, sauces, marinades, and salads.

It is important to choose organic fruits for the peel to avoid chemical residues on the peel. Before use, it is recommended to thoroughly rinse and degrease the zest to remove any possible contamination.

49. Sesame seeds

Sesame is the seed of the sesame indium plant, which can be white, black, or yellow and has a slightly nutty taste and aroma.

Sesame seeds are a popular seasoning that adds texture, aroma and unique flavor to a variety of dishes. They can be used both raw and fried.

Sesame seeds are often added to various sauces, such as tahini (sesame paste sauce), soy sauce, sesame sauces, etc. They give sauces a rich flavor and a light, crunchy texture.

Used for making bread, pastries, sweets, salads, dressings, and as a topping for various dishes.

Sesame seeds can be used to fry meat and fish. Just sprinkle the seeds on the outside or add them to the breading before frying.

You can make sesame oil from them. To do this, they are fried and ground into a paste with the addition of a small amount of vegetable oil.

50. Wild garlic

Wild garlic, also known as wild garlic, has a strong aroma and a pungent taste reminiscent of garlic.

Used for flavoring salads, soups, sauces, and dressings. It is added to soups, stews, and goulash. It is usually added at the end of cooking to preserve its vibrant flavor.

Wild garlic can also be used in a marinade for meat; it adds flavor and pungency, and also helps soften the meat.

You can make a flavored oil from wild garlic by adding the crushed leaves to olive oil and leaving it to steep for several days. This oil can be used for salad dressing.

Chopped wild garlic can be added to a filling for grilled or baked dishes such as potatoes or vegetables. It gives them a rich aroma and taste.